Copyright ©US,

All rights reserved. No part of this book may be reproduced, distributed, or used in any manner whatsoever including photocopying, recording, or other electronic or mechanical methods, without the prior written permission of the publisher, except in the case of brief quotations embodied in critical reviews and certain other noncommercial uses permitted by copyright law.

Table of Contents

Potato Pancakes 5

Mixed Bean Toppings 7

Garden Potato Medley 10

Potato and Kale Soup 13

Garden Vegetable Stew 16

Spicy Red Hummus 19

Harlequin Rice 21

Tex-Mex Pasta 24

Shepherd's Vegetable Pie 27

Potato Boats 31

Fantastic Overnight Cereal 38

Tomato, Corn & Bean Salad 39

Creamy Corn Chowder 41

Bean & Corn Enchiladas 44

Spinach Lasagna 49

Broccomole 56

Chunky Gazpacho 58

Asian Noodles 61

Spaghetti Square Supreme 64

Marinara Surprise 66

Pea Soup 69

Three Bean Salad 72

Nutty Soft Taco 74

Coconut Thai Rice 78

Barbecue Bean Sloppy Joes 82

Crockpot Pizza Potatoes 84

Greta's Gingersnaps with a Twist 86

Simple Split Pea Soup 89

Dal 92

Stove-Top Stew 94

Bean Soup 97

Fried Rice 100

Garbanzo Stew 102

Potato Pancakes

Preparation Time: 20 minutes

Cooking Time: 30 minutes, in batches

Servings: 8

Ingredients

4-5 medium russet potatoes

½ sweet onion

¼ cup water

5 tablespoons white whole wheat flour

¼ cup chopped fresh parsley (optional)

Preparation

Scrub the potatoes and peel the onion. Grate the potatoes and onion together in a food processor. (Or use a box grater, large holes.) Place in a bowl and add the remaining ingredients, mixing well. Preheat oven to 200 degrees. Heat a non-stick griddle until a drop of water bounces off of it. Ladle about 1/3 cup of the potato mixture onto the griddle in batches, flattening slightly. Cook about 5-8 minutes on the first side, then turn and cook an additional 5-8 minutes until golden brown on both sides. Remove to an ovenproof platter and keep warm in the oven until all are cooked. Repeat until all batter is used.

Hint: Unbleached white flour may be substituted for the white whole wheat flour, if desired.

Mixed Bean Toppings

Serve these simple, delicious, dried bean preparations in a variety of ways. They may be cooked on the stove or in a slow cooker, no presoaking is necessary.

Preparation Time: 5 minutes

Cooking Time: 3-4 hours (Slow cooker: 8-10 hours)

Servings: 8

Ingredients

Topping 1:

1 cup split peas

½ cup baby lima beans

½ cup cannellini beans

4 cups water

1 onion, chopped

2 teaspoons basil

1 bay leaf

Topping 2:

1 cup kidney beans

½ cup pinto beans

½ cup cannellini beans

4 cups water

1 onion, chopped

½ teaspoon chili powder

½ teaspoon ground cumin

¼ teaspoon ground oregano

Preparation

Place all ingredients from either 1 or 2 in a large pot. Bring to a boil, reduce heat, cover and cook for 3-4 hours until beans are tender. (In a slow cooker, add all ingredients from either 1 or 2 and cook on high for 8-10 hours.) Serve over brown rice, other whole grains, potatoes, or toast.

Garden Potato Medley

We grew potatoes in our garden this year and there is nothing better tasting than freshly dug potatoes. We also had a huge crop of heirloom tomatoes, and plenty of dinosaur kale (my favorite variety) so this dish is a staple during these fall months.

Preparation Time: 15 minutes

Cooking Time: 20 minutes

Servings: 4

Ingredients

4 cups chunked potatoes

1 tablespoon vegetable broth

1 onion, chopped

1 teaspoon minced fresh garlic

1 jalapeno pepper, seeded and minced

2 ½ cups chopped fresh tomatoes

several twists freshly ground black pepper

4 cups packed chopped dinosaur kale

1 15 ounce can red beans, drained and rinsed

1 tablespoon soy sauce

1 teaspoon chili paste (Sambal Oelek)

¼ cup chopped fresh cilantro

Preparation

Place the potatoes in water to cover, bring to a boil, reduce heat and cook until fairly tender, about 6-8 minutes. Drain and set aside.

Place the vegetable broth in a large non-stick frying pan. Add the onion, garlic and jalapeno. Cook over medium heat, stirring frequently, until vegetables are very soft, about 3-4 minutes. Add tomatoes and black pepper. Cook, uncovered over low heat, stirring occasionally, for 3 minutes. Add the kale and stir gently to combine. Cover and continue to cook for about 2 minutes until kale turns bright green, then add the potatoes and beans. Cook, stirring occasionally for 5 minutes, then add the soy sauce, chili paste and cilantro.

Cook an additional 5 minutes, until kale is tender.

Serve warm or cold.

Hint: Use a variety of tomatoes for an attractive, colorful dish. Use small, new potatoes cooked with the skins on for best flavor. Small red potatoes or a variety of fingerlings are delicious in this recipe. If you can't get dinosaur kale (also called Lacinato Blue), use regular kale, but remove the stems first.

Potato and Kale Soup

Another delicious use for all the potatoes and kale in my garden this year!

Preparation Time: 20 minutes

Cooking Time: 30 minutes

Servings: 6

Ingredients

2 leeks, white and light green parts only, thinly sliced

6 1/3 cups water

6 cups peeled and chopped Yukon Gold potatoes

1 teaspoon dill weed

Freshly ground white pepper to taste

Dash sea salt

4 cups shredded dinosaur kale

1 cup unsweetened almond milk

Preparation

Place the leeks in a large soup pot with 1/3 cup of the water. Cook, stirring occasionally, until leeks soften, about 3-4 minutes. Add the remaining water, the potatoes, dill, pepper and salt. Cover, bring to a boil, reduce heat and cook for about 20 minutes until potatoes are tender. Use an immersion blender to slightly blend the soup, leaving some potato chunks OR remove half of the soup to a blender jar and process until smooth, then return to pot and mix well. Add the dinosaur kale, cook for

5 minutes, then stir in the almond milk and let rest for about 2 minutes before serving.

Hints: Be sure to clean the leeks well before slicing. I usually cut them in half lengthwise before slicing and then rinse them under running water. 6 cups of chopped potatoes is about 3 pounds of potatoes. Dinosaur kale is also called Lacinato Blue and is quite tender. If you can't find it, use regular kale in this recipe but remove the stems first. To shred the kale, roll it slightly, then cut very thin slices (chiffonade).

Garden Vegetable Stew

Preparation Time: 15 minutes

Cooking Time: 30 minutes

Servings: 6-8

1 onion, coarsely chopped

2 cloves garlic, crushed

1 red bell pepper, coarsely chopped

¼ cup vegetable broth

1 28 ounce can fire-roasted chopped tomatoes

4 small zucchini, sliced

2 small yellow crookneck squash, sliced

1 cup cut green beans

1 cup fresh or frozen corn kernels

1 tablespoon soy sauce

1 tablespoon parsley flakes

1 teaspoon dried basil

1 teaspoon dried oregano

1 tablespoon cornstarch mixed in ¼ cup cold water

Preparation

Place the onion, garlic and bell pepper in a large pot with the vegetable broth. Cook and stir until slightly softened, 3 to 4 minutes. Add the tomatoes, zucchini, yellow squash, and beans. Cover and simmer over medium heat for 15 minutes. Add the corn and seasonings, except for the cornstarch mixture. Cook for another 10 minutes. Add the cornstarch mixture and cook, stirring constantly, until thickened.

Hint: If you have some fresh herbs in your garden, use those in place of the dried. Substitute ¼ cup chopped fresh parsley, 1 tablespoon chopped fresh basil and ½ tablespoon chopped fresh oregano.

Spicy Red Hummus

This is a delicious, but spicy, red bell pepper hummus. It has no added tahini or oil, so it is very low in fat, but the flavors just burst in your mouth. Serve as a spread in a wrap or as a dip for baked pita triangles.

Preparation Time: 10 minutes

Chilling Time: 1 hour

Servings: makes about 2 cups

Ingredients

1   15 ounce can garbanzo beans, drained and rinsed

2/3 cup roasted red bell pepper

1/4 cup chopped onion

1 jalapeno, seeded and minced

2-3 cloves garlic, chopped

3 tablespoons cilantro leaves

1 tablespoon chipotle pepper in adobo sauce

1 teaspoon paprika

Several twists freshly ground black pepper

Dash sea salt

1 tablespoon water

Preparation

Place all the ingredients except the water in a food processor and process until quite smooth. Add the water while processing and continue to process until mixture is very smooth. Transfer to a bowl and refrigerate for at least one hour to blend flavors.

Harlequin Rice

Preparation Time: 15 minutes

Cooking Time: 50 minutes

Servings: 4

1 onion, chopped

1 red bell pepper, chopped

1/2 cup chopped green onion

1 teaspoon minced fresh garlic

2 1/4 cups vegetable broth

1 cup uncooked brown basmati rice

1 4 ounce can chopped green chilies

1 4 ounce jar chopped pimientos

1 cup fresh or frozen corn kernels

1 tablespoon parsley flakes

1 teaspoon ground cumin

2 cups packed chopped spinach

1/4 cup chopped fresh cilantro

Freshly ground pepper to taste

Preparation

Place ¼ cup of the vegetable broth in a large pot with the onion, bell pepper, green onion and garlic. Cook, stirring occasionally, until vegetables soften slightly, about 3 minutes. Add the remaining broth, the rice, green chilies, pimientos, corn, parsley and cumin. Cover, bring to a boil, reduce heat and simmer for about 45 minutes until rice is tender. Stir in remaining ingredients and cook for 2 minutes longer.

Tex-Mex Pasta

Preparation Time: 15 minutes

Cooking Time: 20 minutes

Servings: 4

Ingredients

12 ounces whole wheat or brown rice linguine or spaghetti

1 15 ounce can fire-roasted chopped tomatoes

1 15 ounce can kidney beans, drained and rinsed

1 4 ounce can chopped green chilies

1 tablespoon chili powder

1 teaspoon paprika

1 teaspoon ground cumin

½ teaspoon dried oregano

¼ cup water

¼ cup sherry

1 large onion, sliced

½ pound mushrooms, sliced

1 teaspoon minced fresh garlic

1 tablespoon cornstarch mixed in ¼ cup cold water

Preparation

Place a large pot of water on to boil.

Combine the tomatoes, kidney beans, green chilies, chili powder, paprika, cumin and oregano in a bowl and set aside.

Place the water and sherry in a large non-stick sauté pan. Add the onion, mushrooms and garlic and cook, stirring frequently, until the liquid has evaporated, about 15 minutes.

Meanwhile drop the pasta into the boiling water and cook until tender.

Add the tomato mixture to the onions and mushrooms and cook until heated through, about 5 minutes. Add the cornstarch mixture, cook and stir until thickened.

Drain the pasta and place in a bowl. Pour the tomato-vegetable mixture over the pasta and toss gently to mix.

Shepherd's Vegetable Pie

Preparation Time: 35 minutes (need mashed potatoes)

Cooking Time: 1 hour

Servings: 6

Ingredients

3 cups vegetable broth

1 onion, chopped

1 stalk celery, sliced

1 green bell pepper, chopped

½ teaspoon minced bottled fresh garlic

½ teaspoon sage leaves

½ teaspoon marjoram

1 tablespoon soy sauce

1 carrot, thinly sliced

1 ½ cups sliced fresh mushrooms

1 ½ cups cauliflower florets

1 cup thinly sliced cabbage

1 cup green beans, cut in 1 inch pieces

2 tablespoons cornstarch mixed in 1/3 cup cold water

freshly ground pepper to taste

3 cups mashed potatoes

paprika to garnish

Preparation

Preheat oven to 350 degrees.

Place ½ cup of the broth in a large pot with the onion, celery, bell pepper and garlic. Cook, stirring occasionally, for about 4 minutes. Stir in sage, marjoram and soy sauce. Add the remaining vegetable broth and the carrot, mushrooms, cauliflower, cabbage and green beans. Bring to a boil, cover, reduce heat and cook for 20 minutes, stirring occasionally. Add the cornstarch mixture and stir until thickened. Season with pepper to taste. Transfer to a casserole dish. Cover vegetable mixture with mashed potatoes and sprinkle with paprika. Bake for 30 minutes until potatoes are slightly browned.

Hint: Thin the mashed potatoes with a little soy milk or vegetable broth if they are too stiff to spread. Put them in a bowl, add a small amount of the liquid and beat by hand or with an electric beater until they are spreadable.

Potato Boats

Servings: 5

Preparation Time: 15 minutes

Cooking Time: 1 ¼ hours

Ingredients

5 large baking potatoes

1 ½ cups soymilk

1 cup each: frozen peas, corn, lima beans, thawed

¾ cup grated soy cheese

paprika

Preparation

Preheat oven to 475 degrees.

Scrub potatoes and prick all over with a fork. Place on medium oven rack. Bake for about 1 hour until tender.

Thaw frozen vegetables under cool water and drain. Set aside.

Remove potatoes from oven. Cut off a small portion of the top lengthwise and scrape off excess potato from the skin. Discard top. Scoop out potato center from the remaining part of the potato, leaving a small edge next to the skin. Reserve.

Reduce oven heat to 350 degrees.

Place the potato centers in a bowl and mash with a potato masher or electric beater, adding a small amount of soymilk at a time, until smooth. Stir in vegetables and soy cheese. Place the potato mixture back into the potato shells, mounding it as high as necessary to use all of the mixture. Place on a baking sheet. Sprinkle with paprika. Bake for 15 minutes, then broil on low for 2-3 minutes to brown slightly.

Serve plain or with a gravy or sauce.

Hint: These potatoes reheat well. Great for lunch or a snack. For less servings, reduce the amount of potatoes, vegetables and soymilk accordingly.

The following recipe is by Heather McDougall. It is a delicious way to use potatoes and parsnips for a creamy, earthy soup. Many people are unfamiliar with parsnips. They can be found in your produce section and they look like carrots except they are white in color.

Potato and Parsnip Soup

Servings 4-6

Preparation Time: 20 minutes

Cooking Time(without garlic): 35 minutes

Cooking Time (with garlic): 45 minutes

Ingredients

6 cups vegetable broth

1 onion chopped

4 medium parsnips, peeled and cubed

2 large Russet potatoes, peeled and cubed

1 carrot, peeled and sliced

1 tablespoon lemon juice

salt and pepper to taste

1 tablespoon chopped fresh parsley

Preparation

Saute onion in ½ cup vegetable broth until soft, about 5 minutes. Add remaining broth, parsnips, potatoes, and carrot. Bring to a boil, reduce to simmer, and cook for 25 minutes, or until all vegetables are soft. Turn off heat and prepare to puree soup. Using a blender, puree small amounts of soup at a time and transfer to another medium saucepan. When finished, heat soup on low for 5 minutes stirring occasionally. Remove from heat, add lemon juice, and salt and pepper to taste.

Roasted Garlic Bread

Preparation Time: 5 minutes

Roasting Time: 45 minutes

Ingredients

1 baguette, sliced on the diagonal

1 head garlic

4 tablespoons vegetable broth

salt to taste

Preparation

Preheat oven to 400 degrees. Cut top of garlic head off and drizzle 2 tablespoons of broth over the top. Wrap in parchment paper, then wrap in foil and place in oven for 45 minutes. Remove from oven and let cool. Place bread in oven on a baking sheet and bake until light brown. Watch carefully. Squeeze out garlic from cloves, add remaining broth and salt, and mix until smooth. Spread on toasted bread.

Fantastic Overnight Cereal

This is a simple way to make a delicious, healthy breakfast by preparing it the night before so it will be ready to eat in the morning. John says this is the best oatmeal ever!

Preparation Time: 5 minutes

Cooking Time: none

Servings: 1

Ingredients

1 cup old fashioned organic rolled oats

1 cup soy or rice milk, apple juice, or water

1 tablespoon currants or raisins

½ teaspoon cinnamon

Ingredients

Combine all ingredients in a container and mix well. Cover and refrigerate overnight.

The next morning either enjoy the cereal cold or microwave until warmed. Serve with sliced bananas or seasonal fresh berries sprinkled over the top.

Tomato, Corn & Bean Salad

Preparation Time: 15 minutes

Resting Time: 15 minutes

Servings: 4

Ingredients

1 cup fresh, frozen (thawed), or canned corn kernels

2 cups diced tomatoes

1 red onion, diced

2 red, yellow, orange, or green bell pepper, diced

1 tablespoon chopped fresh basil

1 can white beans (great northern, cannellini, navy), drained and rinsed

1 tablespoon fresh lime juice

1 teaspoon rice vinegar

salt, to taste

In a large bowl, combine all of the ingredients and set aside for 15 minutes or more to allow the flavors to develop. Add salt and serve at room temperature.

Creamy Corn Chowder

This recipe was sent in by a subscriber and it is a delicious way to use some of the fresh corn that is available now. Lydia says it may also be made with frozen corn.

Preparation Time: 30 minutes

Cooking Time: 45 minutes

Servings: 6-8

Ingredients

2 ½ cups diced potatoes, cooked

2/3 cup finely chopped white onion

4 ½ cups vegetable broth

5 cups fresh sweet corn (off the cob), 7-8 cobs

2 bay leaves

¼ teaspoon rosemary, slightly crushed

¼ teaspoon thyme, slightly crushed

salt and pepper to taste

Preparation

Cook the potatoes in water to cover until tender, about 10 minutes. Drain and set aside.

Place the onion in ½ cup of the vegetable broth and cook, stirring occasionally, for about 5 minutes. Add 3 cups of the corn and ½ cup more of the broth and cook for another 5 minutes. Add 2 more cups of broth, bring to a boil, reduce heat and simmer for 20 minutes. Transfer in batches to a blender jar and process until smooth. Return to pot, add the cooked potatoes, the remaining vegetable broth and corn, and the bay leaves, rosemary and thyme. Return to boil, reduce heat, cover and simmer for about 10 minutes. Remove bay leaves, season to taste and serve hot.

Hint: If you have an immersion blender the soup can be blended right in the cooking pot (as long as you are not using a non-stick pot because you might damage the coating) and eliminate the step of transferring the soup to a blender jar.

Bean & Corn Enchiladas

This is another variation on our favorite enchiladas. I make these often when I have leftover pinto beans from our usual bean burrito meal. We like all the ingredients inside the enchiladas, so it is very easy if you just mix the ingredients together and then spread the mixture on the tortilla.

Preparation Time: 40 minutes

Cooking Time: 45 minutes

Servings: 6-8

Ingredients

Sauce:

2   8 ounce cans tomato sauce

3   cups water

4 tablespoons cornstarch

3 tablespoons chili powder

½ teaspoon onion powder

¼ teaspoon garlic powder

Preparation

Place all ingredients for the sauce in a saucepan. Mix well with a whisk until well combined. Cook and stir over medium heat until thickened, about 5 minutes. Taste and add more chili powder if desired. Set aside.

10 whole wheat tortillas

4 cups mashed pinto beans

1 cup chopped green onions

1 ½ cups frozen corn kernels, thawed

1 2.25 ounce can sliced ripe olives, drained

1-2 tablespoons chopped green chilies (optional)

grated soy cheese (optional)

Preparation

Preheat oven to 350 degrees.

To assemble casserole:

Place the beans in a large bowl. Add the onions, corn, olives and green chilies (if you wish). Mix gently until well combined.

Place 1½ cups of the sauce in the bottom of a large non-stick oblong baking dish. Take 1 tortilla at a time and spread a line of the bean mixture down the center of the tortilla. Roll up and place seam side down in the baking dish. Repeat with remaining tortillas, placing them snugly next to each other. Pour the rest of the sauce over the rolled up tortillas, spreading it out evenly. Sprinkle a small amount of grated soy cheese over the top, if desired. Cover with parchment paper, then cover with aluminum foil, crimping the edges over the baking dish. Bake for 45 minutes. Remove from oven and let rest for about 5 minutes before cutting. Serve with salsa and tofu sour cream, if desired.

Variation: This may also be made with corn tortillas instead of the wheat tortillas. You will need about 15-16 corn tortillas. The remaining directions remain the same.

Spinach Lasagna

This is our old favorite lasagna recipe, but I have changed the kind of tofu used to the recipe for tofu ricotta from Alex Bury found in a previous newsletter. We like this version even better because of the creamy consistency of the tofu filling. I also like to make this with fresh spinach instead of frozen.

Preparation Time: 40 minutes

Cooking Time: 60 minutes

Resting Time: 10 minutes

Servings: 6-8

Ingredients

Prepare the ricotta before assembling the lasagna.

Tofu Ricotta:

1 12.3 ounce package silken tofu

1 pound fresh water-packed firm tofu

2 teaspoons minced garlic

¼ cup nutritional yeast

½ teaspoon salt

½ teaspoon pepper

1 tablespoon parsley flakes

1 teaspoon basil

1 teaspoon oregano

¼ cup lemon juice

¼ cup soy milk

Preparation

Combine all of the above ingredients in a food processor and process until fairly smooth. Refrigerate until ready to use.

Lasagna:

1 recipe Tofu Ricotta

1-2 bags fresh, washed spinach

8 ounces lasagna noodles

7 cups fat-free pasta sauce

12 ounces Soy mozzarella cheese, grated

¼ cup soy parmesan cheese

Place the tofu ricotta into a large bowl. Set aside.

Bring a large pot of water to a boil. Drop in the lasagna noodles, stir, cook uncovered until just softened. Do not overcook. Remove from water and drain, hanging them up to dry slightly. OR use the no-boil lasagna noodles and eliminate this step entirely.

Prepare the spinach next. Use at least 1 bag, 2 if you really like spinach. Steam the fresh spinach just until slightly wilted (about a minute or two), drain well, then either mix the spinach into the tofu ricotta or layer the spinach over the tofu ricotta in 2 batches before sprinkling with the grated soy cheese. (See assembly directions below.)

Preheat oven to 350 degrees.

Lightly oil the bottom of a 9x13 inch baking dish. (Remove any excess oil with a paper towel.) Place 1 cup of the pasta sauce in the bottom of the baking dish and smooth over the bottom. Place 1 layer of the noodles over the sauce. Then add half of the tofu mixture and smooth out. Sprinkle half of the soy cheese over that, then spread 2 cups more of the sauce over the cheese. Add another layer of noodles, the rest of the tofu mixture, the remaining cheese, 2 cups more of the sauce, and the rest of the noodles. Spoon the remaining 2 cups of sauce over the noodles (make sure you cover all the edges), sprinkle some soy parmesan over the top. Cover with parchment paper and then cover with foil. Bake for 60 minutes. Remove from oven and let rest for 10 minutes before cutting.

Variation: This may be made with frozen spinach. Use a 10 ounce box (or more) and thaw in a colander. Drain well and press out any excess water with your hands. Mix into the tofu ricotta before assembling lasagna.

Hints: This may be prepared ahead of time and refrigerated before baking. Add about 15 minutes to the baking time.

Place the corn in a saucepan with 1/3 cup water. Bring to a boil, reduce heat, cover and cook about 5 minutes, until corn is tender. Remove from heat and let cool slightly. Pour into a food processor and process until smooth. Gradually add the broth while processing and continue until soup is quite smooth. Return to saucepan, heat through and serve.

Broccomole

This makes a great substitute for guacamole (I know it sounds a bit strange!). Try it with baked chips for dipping, or use on burritos or tacos.

Preparation Time: 20 minutes

Chilling Time: 2 hours

Servings: Makes 2 cups

Ingredients

1 ½ cups broccoli stems

1 ½ tablespoons lemon juice

¼ teaspoon cumin

1/8 teaspoon garlic powder

1 tomato, diced

1-2 green onions, chopped

¼ cup chopped green chilies

¼ cup chopped cilantro (optional)

Preparation

Peel broccoli stems, chop into pieces, and steam until tender, about 10 minutes. Place in a food processor and blend broccoli stems with lemon juice, cumin and garlic powder until completely smooth. Place in a bowl, add remaining ingredients and mix well. Chill before serving.

Chunky Gazpacho

During the summer months I always serve several different versions of gazpacho, the classic cold tomato soup. This one requires a lot of chopped vegetables, so it takes a bit longer to prepare. (See hint below.) It will keep for several days in the refrigerator and makes a great meal on those days when it is too hot to cook.

Preparation Time: 20-40 minutes

Chilling Time: 3-4 hours

Servings:10

Ingredients

4 cups tomato juice

2 cups peeled, seeded and chopped tomatoes

1 cup chopped cucumber

1/2 cup chopped red onion

1/2 cup chopped celery

1/2 cup corn kernels

1/2 cup chopped green pepper

1/4 cup chopped green onions

1/4 cup chopped zucchini

1/4 cup chopped green chilies (canned)

1/4 cup chopped fresh parsley

1/4 cup chopped cilantro (optional)

1-2 cloves garlic, minced

2 tablespoons red wine vinegar

2 tablespoons lime juice

1 tablespoon hot sauce (like Tabasco), optional

Preparation

Combine all the ingredients in a large bowl. Cover and chill for several hours before serving.

Hint: The ingredients may be prepared by using a food processor. This is a great time saver. This may also be prepared by pureeing half of the ingredients and leaving the remaining ingredients finely chopped.

Note: To peel tomatoes, use one of the new serrated peelers, or dip briefly in boiling water until the skins loosen, then just slip the skins off.

Asian Noodles

Preparation Time: 20 minutes

Cooking Time: 20 minutes

Servings: 4

Ingredients

½ cup water

1-2 cloves garlic, crushed

1 teaspoon fresh grated ginger

1/8 - 1/4 teaspoon crushed red pepper flakes

2 carrots, shredded

1 medium bunch broccoli, cut into florets

1/2 lb mushrooms, sliced

1 bunch green onions, cut in 1 inch pieces

1/4 cup soy sauce

½ pound soba noodles

Preparation

1 tablespoon cornstarch mixed with 2 tablespoons cold water.

Place garlic, ginger, red pepper, carrots and broccoli in a wok or large pan with the 1/2 cup water and 2 tablespoons of the soy sauce. Cook and stir for 5 minutes. Add mushrooms and green onions. Cook, stirring occasionally, for about 10 minutes.

Meanwhile prepare the soba noodles according to package directions. Drain. Toss with the remaining soy sauce. Set aside.

Mix cornstarch with water. Add to vegetable mixture, cook and stir until thickened. Pour over soba noodles and mix well. Serve at room temperature, or refrigerate and serve cold.

Spaghetti Square Supreme

Look for spaghetti squash in the produce section of your market. It is a creamy yellow color, oblong shaped, and when cooked, the strands pull out like cooked spaghetti. It is very low in calories and makes an excellent substitute for cooked pasta.

Preparation Time: 5 minutes

Cooking Time: variable

Servings: 6-8

Ingredients

1 spaghetti squash

Preparation (Methods)

1) Leave whole and prick the skin all over with the tines of a fork. Bake in a 350 degree oven for about 1 hour. Cut in half at once to stop the cooking process. Let cool briefly, then remove seeds. Rake the strands out with a fork.

2) Cut squash in half and remove the seeds. Place cut side down in a baking dish and bake for about 45 minutes. Turn over and rake out the cooked strands with a fork.

3) Cut squash in half and remove the seeds. Microwave for 10-15 minutes, cut side up in a

baking dish with a small amount of water in the bottom. Rake out cooked strands with a fork.

4) Cut squash in half and remove the seeds. Place in a large steamer pot with about 2 inches of water covering the bottom. Cover and steam for about 30 minutes. Rake out cooked strands with a fork.

Serve the spaghetti squash with your favorite low fat marinara sauce for a delicious weight-loss meal. Or try the following delicious topping for your spaghetti squash.

Marinara Surprise

Preparation Time: 15 minutes

Cooking Time: 45 minutes

Servings: 6

Ingredients

½ cup water

1 onion, chopped

½ cup chopped celery

½ cup chopped carrot

2-3 cloves minced garlic

1 15 ounce can chopped fire-roasted tomatoes

1 15 ounce can pinto beans, drained and rinsed

2 teaspoon basil

2 teaspoons chili powder

1 teaspoon paprika

Preparation

2 cups packed, chopped, fresh Swiss chard

Place the water in a large pot. Add the onion, celery, carrot and garlic. Cook, stirring occasionally, until vegetables soften slightly. Add the tomatoes, beans and seasonings.

Reduce heat and cook, covered, for 30 minutes. Add the chard and cook for an additional 10 minutes.

Hints: Use any variety of cooked beans that you wish for variation. If you can't find the fire roasted tomatoes, use plain chopped tomatoes.

Pea Soup

This is my family's favorite pea soup. I have been making this version for over 25 years. This tastes even better the next day and it is great over baked potatoes, too!

Preparation Time: 15 minutes

Cooking Time: 2 hours

Servings: 8-10

Ingredients

1 cup green split peas

½ cup dried baby lima beans

¼ cup barley

8 cups water

1 onion, chopped

2 bay leaves

1 teaspoon celery seed

2 cups vegetable broth

2 carrots, chopped

2 potatoes, chunked

2 celery stalks, chopped

2 tablespoons parsley flakes

1 teaspoon basil

1 teaspoon paprika

1/8 teaspoon white pepper

freshly ground black pepper to taste

Preparation

Place split peas, lima beans, barley and water in a large pot. Bring to a boil, reduce heat and add bay leaves and celery seed. Cover and cook over low heat for 1 hour. Add remaining ingredients and cook for an additional 1 hour.

Hints: If you want to make this without the lima beans, increase the split peas to 2 cups and reduce the initial cooking time to ½ hour. This freezes well and reheats well. For a delicious smoky flavor, try adding a couple drops of liquid smoke to the soup about 15 minutes before the end of the cooking time.

Three Bean Salad

This is a very fast and easy salad. Great to have on hand in your refrigerator for a quick snack. It also packs well so it is easy to take with you to work. This can be made as mild or as spicy as you like it by changing the kind of salsa used.

Preparation Time: 15 minutes

Chilling Time: at least 1 hour

Servings: 6

Ingredients

1   15 ounce can black beans, drained and rinsed

1   15 ounce can kidney beans, drained and rinsed

1   15 ounce can garbanzo beans, drained and rinsed

1 small, mild, sweet onion, thinly sliced

2 stalks celery, sliced

1 tomato, chopped

1 cup salsa, mild, medium, or hot

2 tablespoons lime juice

1 teaspoon chili powder (optional)

Preparation

Combine beans and vegetables in a large bowl. Place the salsa in a small container, then add the lime juice and chili powder. Stir or shake to combine. Pour over the bean mixture and toss to mix. Refrigerate at least 1 hour to allow flavors to blend.

Nutty Soft Taco

I have been making these tacos for my family for over 25 years. This recipe makes enough for dinner and leftovers for a couple of lunches. The filling may also be frozen for later use. We consider this a richer food because of the nuts used, so I usually only make it once or twice a year. Toppings for the tacos may be varied according to your tastes.

Preparation Time: 15 minutes

Cooking Time: 15 minutes

Servings: makes about 3 cups

Ingredients

Filling:

¾ cup roasted unsalted peanuts

½ cup raw sunflower seeds

½ cup roasted sunflower seeds

½ cup sesame seeds

1 teaspoon cumin seeds

½ to 1 cup water

1 6 ounce can tomato paste

soft corn tortillas

Toppings:

chopped green onions

chopped tomatoes

shredded lettuce

alfalfa sprouts

salsa

Preparation

Place the peanuts and raw sunflower seeds in a saucepan with water to cover. Cover and cook for 15 minutes. Drain off remaining water and reserve. Place the cooked peanuts and sunflower seeds in a food processor. Add the roasted sunflower seeds, the sesame seeds, the cumin seeds and about ½ cup of the reserved cooking water. (Add more water if necessary to reach ½ cup.) Process until blended. Add the tomato paste and process until well blended. Add more water, a small amount at a time, until mixture is a spreadable consistency. Serve warm or cold. Place a line of the filling down the center of the tortilla, layer on the toppings and salsa of your choice, roll up and eat.

Hints: Store unused nuts and seeds in the freezer so they don't spoil.

Coconut Thai Rice

This is a delicious variation on the Thai Green Curry Rice from last month's newsletter.

Print out the recipe from last month and make these substitutions.

In place of the ½ cup soy sauce, use only 1 tablespoon. Mix 1 ½ teaspoons of coconut extract into 1 ½ cups rice or almond milk, and stir this into the vegetable mixture. Use cooked Thai purple rice in place of the cooked brown rice. All other ingredients remain the same.

Coconut extract in rice or almond milk makes a wonderful substitution for coconut milk in recipes.

Preparation Time: 15 minutes

Cooking Time: 15 minutes

Servings: 2-4

Preparation

¼ cup water

1-2 zucchini, diced

1 carrot, grated

2 shallots, diced

3 cups vegetable broth

1 cup orzo

pinch of curry powder

pinch of salt

several twists of freshly ground pepper

¼ cup soy parmesan cheese

Preparation

Place the water in a large non-stick frying pan. Add the zucchini, carrot and shallots. Cook, stirring occasionally until softened, about 4-5 minutes. Add the vegetable broth and bring to a boil. Stir in the orzo and curry powder. Cook until orzo is tender, about 5-6 minutes. Stir in the salt, pepper and soy parmesan. Cook for another minute and serve hot.

Hint: One of the best tasting soy parmesan cheese substitutes on the market is made by The Vegetarian Express. It is called Parma Zaan Sprinkles.

Barbecue Bean Sloppy Joes

Preparation Time: 10 minutes (need cooked rice)

Cooking time: 15 minutes

Servings: 6-8

Ingredients

1 onion, chopped

1 bell pepper, chopped

¼ cup vegetable broth

3 cups cooked brown rice

2 15 ounce cans pinto beans, undrained

¾ cup fat-free barbecue sauce

1 ½ tablespoons chili powder

whole wheat buns

Preparation

Place the onion and bell pepper in a non-stick pan with the vegetable broth. Cook, stirring occasionally until vegetables soften slightly, about 3 minutes. Add remaining ingredients (except the buns) and cook for about 12 minutes, until well heated.

Hints: There are many delicious barbecue sauces on the market shelves these days. Choose one without oil and preferably without high fructose corn syrup. Use another kind of bean to vary the recipe, or maybe one can each of pinto and black or white. There are several manufacturers that make frozen cooked whole grain brown rice that reheats in the microwave in 3 minutes.

Crockpot Pizza Potatoes

Preparation Time: 20 minutes

Cooking Time: 6-8 hours on LOW

Servings: 6-8

 Ingredient

4 cups thinly sliced potatoes (use a Mandolin for best results)

2-3 cups of pizza toppings

Sliced onion

Sliced mushrooms

Sliced bell peppers

Sliced tomatoes

Sliced water-packed artichoke hearts

Sliced black olives

Fresh spinach

2 15 ounce cans fat-free pizza sauce or Marinara sauce

¼ cup water

Preparation

Mix the water into the sauce and set aside.

Place 2 cups of the potatoes in the bottom of the crockpot. Layer all of the toppings that you choose to include over the potatoes. Cover with half of the sauce. Layer on the remaining 2 cups of potatoes and finish with the sauce. Cover and cook on low for 6-8 hours.

Greta's Gingersnaps with a Twist

Ingredients

In a medium bowl sift:

2 cups whole wheat pastry flour

1 teaspoon ginger (ground)

1 teaspoon cloves (ground)

1 teaspoon cinnamon (ground)

1/2 teaspoon salt

2 teaspoons baking soda

In a large bowl mix:

1/4 cup + 2 tablespoons Wonderslim Fat & Egg Substitute

1 cup Sucanat

1 ½ tablespoons water

1/4 cup molasses (Grandma's is my favorite!)

Preparation

Add the dry ingredients to the wet and mix thoroughly. Chill the dough before handling further.

Pre-heat oven to 350 degrees and line cookie sheet with parchment paper or use a non stick pan.

Roll dough into small (1") balls (a melon baller works good)

Sprinkle some sugar or Sucanat on a plate and roll the balls in it. Place 2 inches apart on the prepared cookie sheet and bake at 350 for about 10 minutes (cookies will puff and then collapse). Let rest for a minute or 2 and remove to a cooling rack.

Simple Split Pea Soup

You will likely have the ingredients for this tasty soup already in your cupboards and pantry, so no need for an extra trip to the market for supplies.

Preparation Time: 15 minutes

Cooking Time: 1 hour

Resting Time: 15 minutes (optional for thickening)

Servings: 10

Ingredients

2 cups green split peas

8 cups water

1 onion, chopped

2 carrots, chopped

2 stalks celery, chopped

2-3 potatoes, chunked

2 bay leaves

2 tablespoons parsley flakes

1 tablespoon Dijon-style mustard

1 teaspoon basil

1 teaspoon paprika

¼ teaspoon black pepper

Preparation

Place the peas and water in a large soup pot. Bring to a boil, reduce heat and simmer uncovered for 20 minutes. Add the remaining ingredients, mix well and bring to a boil again. Reduce heat, cover and simmer for about 40 minutes, until vegetables are tender. Remove from heat and let rest for 15 minutes to thicken before serving, if desired. Season with a bit of sea salt before serving (optional).

Hints: This will thicken even more as it cools, and will be very thick if refrigerated until the next day. This is wonderful in a bowl with some fresh baked bread, or ladle it over baked potatoes or brown rice.

Variation: For a delicious Curried Split Pea Soup, leave out all of the seasonings in the above recipe and add 2-3 tablespoons curry powder and ¼ cup nutritional yeast.

Dal

This simple, economical spread of split peas or mung beans has been one of our favorites for more than thirty years.

Preparation Time: 2 minutes

Cooking Time: 1 hour

Resting Time: 15 minutes

Servings: 8-10

2 cups split mung beans, chana dal or yellow split peas

5 cups water

1 ½ tablespoons curry powder (sweet, mild or spicy)

Preparation

Place the beans or peas and the water in a medium pot. Bring to a boil, reduce heat, cover and simmer for 30 minutes. Add the curry powder, mix well and cook uncovered for 30 minutes longer. Transfer to a serving bowl and let rest for about 15 minutes, to thicken slightly, before serving.

Hints: Serve rolled up in a corn or flour tortilla with toppings of your choice. I like them plain, while John usually tops his with some Sriracha sauce. Or try this Dal over baked potatoes or rice. It also makes a delicious sandwich spread when cold.

Stove-Top Stew

Serve this simple, hearty stew over a large mound of brown rice or any other choice of whole grains.

Preparation Time: 10 minutes

Cooking Time: 45 minutes

Servings: 4

Ingredients

¼ cup water

1 onion, chopped

½ teaspoon minced garlic

2 carrots, sliced

2 stalks celery, sliced

2-3 potatoes, chunked

1 15 ounce can tomato sauce

1 tablespoon soy sauce

1 tablespoon parsley flakes

½ teaspoon paprika

½ teaspoon basil

½ teaspoon chili powder

¼ teaspoon dry mustard

¼ teaspoon ground cumin

¼ teaspoon black pepper

1 cup chopped spinach, kale or chard (optional)

Preparation

Place the water in a pot with the onion, garlic, carrots, celery and potatoes. Cook, stirring occasionally, for 10 minutes. Add the remaining ingredients, except for the greens. Bring to a boil, reduce heat, cover and cook for 30 minutes, until all vegetables are tender. Stir in the greens, if desired, and cook until tender, between 2-5 minutes.

Hints: Other vegetables may be added as desired, such as zucchini and/or mushrooms. Add these with the remaining ingredients. If you use vegetables that are in season, and local, this stew is a very economical meal.

Bean Soup

This is a basic soup recipe that can be made with any type of dried beans. I first stared making it with Great Northern beans, but have used Soldier, Cranberry, Scarlet Runner, Red Calypso, Steuben Yellow Eyes, Rattlesnake, and Christmas as well as other heirloom beans in this recipe. Vary the seasonings to suit your own tastes. Beans and vegetables make this a stick-to-your-ribs meal

Preparation Time: 10 minutes

Cooking Time: 3-4 hours (Slow cooker: 8-10 hours)

Servings: 8

Ingredients

2 cups dried beans

8 cups water

2 onions, chopped

2-4 stalks celery, chopped

2 bay leaves

½ teaspoon sage

½ teaspoon oregano

2 tablespoons low sodium soy sauce

Preparation

Place all ingredients in a large pot and bring to a boil. Reduce heat, cover and simmer for 3-4 hours until beans are tender. (In a slow cooker, this will take about 8-10 hours on high.)

Fried Rice

This is a delicious way to use leftover brown rice. Pick any vegetables that are in season and reasonably priced at the market.

Preparation Time: 15 minutes (need cooked rice)

Cooking Time: 15 minutes

Servings: 6

Ingredients

¼ cup water

½-1 teaspoon crushed garlic

½-1 teaspoon grated ginger

6 cups mixed chopped vegetables

4 cups cooked brown rice

¼ cup low sodium soy sauce

Preparation

Place the water in a wok or large non-stick frying pan. Add the garlic and ginger and heat until water boils. Add the vegetables and cook, stirring frequently, until vegetables are crisp tender. Stir in the rice and soy sauce. Cook until heated through, about 2 minutes.

Hints: Use a variety of vegetables for color and flavor. Some examples are: carrots, broccoli, red peppers, green onions, celery, snow peas, bok choy, etc. Cut them into uniform sizes so they all cook in about the same length of time.

Garbanzo Stew

This is another of our old favorites, made with inexpensive pantry staples. Make it on the stove or in a slow cooker. Garbanzo beans require a long cooking time to be really tender, so plan accordingly.

Preparation Time: 15 minutes (overnight soaking needed)

Cooking Time: 4 hours (Slow cooker: 8-10 hours)

Servings: 10

Ingredients

2 cups uncooked garbanzo beans (chick peas)

8-10 cups water

2 potatoes, chunked

2 carrots, thickly sliced

2 stalks celery, thickly sliced

2 onions, chopped

2 tablespoons low sodium soy sauce

Preparation

Soak the garbanzos overnight in water to cover. Drain. Place the garbanzos and 8 cups water in a large pot. Bring to a boil, reduce heat, cover and cook for 2 hours. Add remaining ingredients and cook an additional 2 hours, adding more water if necessary.

Hints: To make in a slow cooker, combine the soaked, drained beans with the remaining ingredients (use only 8 cups of water) and cook for 8-10 hours on high.

Made in the USA
Middletown, DE
30 September 2020